TRACHEOSTOMY MANAGEMENT

Made Simple For The Head And Neck Cancer Patient

Kara Mosesso, ANP-BC

Elizabeth Von Euw, MS, CCC-SLP

Miriam O'Leary, MD

Richard O. Wein, MD, FACS

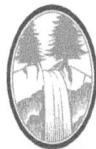

**PROVENIR
PUBLISHING**

Spokane, Washington

www.provenirpublishing.com

Tracheostomy Management: Made Simple for the Head and Neck Cancer Patient

Published by Provenir Publishing, LLC, P. O. Box 211, Greenacres, WA 99016-0211

Production Credits

Lead Editor: Richard Wein

Editor: Steve Hanson

Art Director and Illustration: Micah Harman

Cover Design: Micah Harman

Printing History: April 2014, First Edition.

Contents

Introduction

If you received this book, you or a loved one probably have been diagnosed with head and neck cancer and have been told by your physician that you may need a tracheostomy. The word tracheostomy often evokes feelings of fear and anxiety in patients. The thought of a hole in the front of the neck is overwhelming, especially in connection with a cancer diagnosis. It is hard to imagine returning to a normal life after this procedure, and contemplating the care required can be daunting. These concerns are natural. However, while having a tracheostomy can be life altering, it is not debilitating.

The tracheotomy procedure is performed fairly commonly in head and neck cancer patients. In this procedure, a hole is surgically created in the front of the neck and into the trachea (windpipe) to establish an airway in the neck. This hole, or stoma, is referred to as a tracheostomy. Once the stoma is created, it is maintained by inserting a tracheostomy tube.

Becoming informed about the initial procedure and management of your tracheostomy will help alleviate your anxieties and fears. That is the objective of this handbook. It will assist in the transition from the hospital to home and provide you with information you will need to manage your tracheostomy appropriately.

Part One

Indications And Technique

The purpose of a tracheostomy is to create a "bypass route" for the airway. The tracheostomy transitions the primary route of the airway from the mouth and nose to the neck. If there is an anticipated obstruction of the upper airway due to disease (progressing infection or tumor) or a proposed surgical procedure, a tracheostomy is a reasonable consideration to provide a stable, safe airway.

Patients requiring intubation* with an anticipated prolonged need for ventilatory assistance in an Intensive Care Unit (ICU) may also require tracheostomy placement. In this setting, the tracheostomy may be used to improve patient comfort. Importantly, it can help the process of weaning the patient from the ventilator while decreasing the risk of long-term airway trauma and scarring that can result from prolonged intubation.

*Transoral breathing tube placed to stabilize the airway in an emergency or in the operating room at the time of surgery.

More commonly, a tracheostomy is performed at the time of a patient's surgery for a head and neck cancer. Many of these surgeries can cause significant swelling in the mouth and throat. This may temporarily compromise a patient's airway. To alleviate this, your physician may recommend a temporary tracheostomy tube which can be removed once the swelling from surgery subsides and it is determined that you have a safe airway.

Sometimes a patient is treated with radiation instead of, or in addition to, surgery. Radiation can also cause edema (swelling) in the throat which may be severe enough to require a temporary tracheostomy.

The size, location, and rate of growth of a tumor will determine whether or not a tracheostomy may be necessary. In addition, the health of the patient is a factor. For example a tracheostomy may be necessary for patients who have difficulty swallowing, significant weight loss and/or malnutrition, multiple medical problems (such as chronic heart and/or lung diseases), or are at an advanced age.

> Although infrequent, patients may require an emergent tracheostomy if they develop acute respiratory distress because of the progression of their tumor.

A tracheostomy may also be recommended for patients having difficulty tolerating or aspirating (inhaling) their secretions. These challenges can come because of pain associated with the tumor, difficulty swallowing, vocal cord paralysis, or altered nerve function as a side effect of the tumor or treatment. A tracheostomy can assist with "pulmonary toilet" so that secretions can be suctioned through the tracheostomy to clear the airway.

Part Two

Technique For Placement

Tracheostomy is typically done with an open surgical technique and may be performed in the operating room or ICU. Patients are under general anesthesia with the placement of an endotracheal tube to stabilize the airway prior to the start of the procedure. In the event of an acute airway emergency, when intubation is not possible, "awake" tracheostomy with the use of local anesthesia (similar to Novocaine) may also be performed.

At the time of tracheostomy, a horizontal incision is made at the central lower neck. The soft tissues and muscle are divided to create a path to the trachea where a small window in the trachea is created for insertion of the tracheostomy tube. *(See fig. 1 on page 8)* In some cases, percutaneous tracheostomy tube placement is done. This is most commonly performed in an ICU setting and involves placement of a tracheostomy tube without a formal incision and utilizes a technique that is similar to the placement of an intravenous catheter.

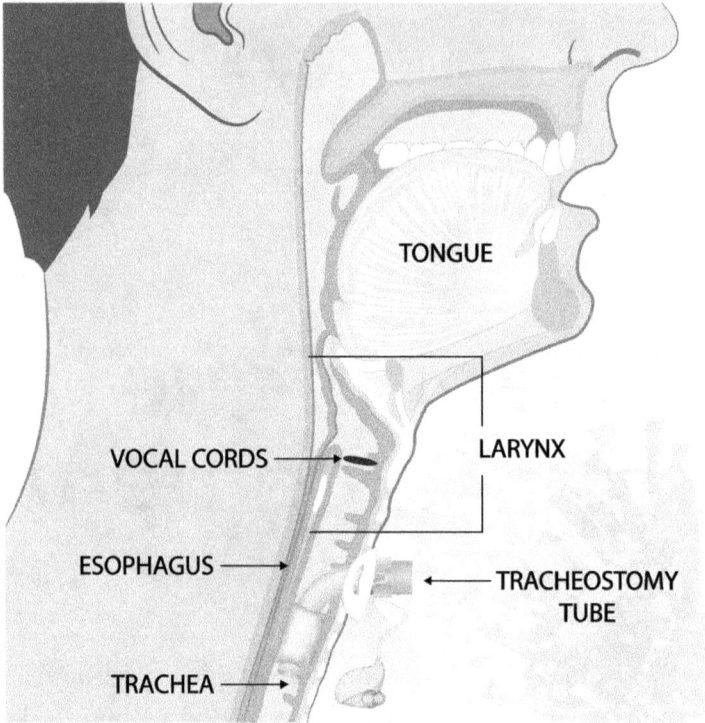

fig. 1

TONGUE

VOCAL CORDS ——→

LARYNX

ESOPHAGUS ——→

TRACHEOSTOMY
TUBE

TRACHEA ——→

*Sagittal view of lateral neck demonstrating the location of tracheos-
tomy placement relative to surrounding anatomy.*

As with any surgical procedure, tracheostomy carries some risk. Short-term complications can include bleeding, infection, damage to the trachea, subcutaneous emphysema (air trapped in tissue under the skin of the neck), or pneumothorax (build-up of air between the chest wall and lungs causing pain, breathing problems, or lung collapse).

Long-term complications are more likely the longer the tracheostomy is in place. These include displacement of the tracheostomy tube from the trachea, narrowing of the trachea, abnormal tissue formation in the trachea (granulation tissue), obstruction of the tracheostomy tube, difficulty swallowing, infection, and development of a passage between the trachea and esophagus known as a tracheoesophageal fistula.

A rare long-term complication is a trachea-innominate fistula, in which the tracheostomy tube erodes through the tracheal wall into a large blood vessel called the innominate artery.

Part Three

Types Of Tracheostomy Tubes

Tracheostomy tubes may be semi-flexible plastic, rigid plastic or metal. **Metal tubes** are not commonly used. **Plastic tracheostomy tubes** are typically used for initial tube placement. All tracheostomy tubes have an outer cannula with a baseplate (flange) that rests against the neck. There are slits on each side of the flange for a tracheostomy tie to help hold the tube in place. An obturator is used to help with tracheostomy tube insertion. It fits inside the outer cannula and has a rounded end to guide tube insertion. The obturator is removed once the tube is placed. *(See fig. 2 on page 13)*

A tracheostomy tube can have a single or dual cannula. A dual cannula tube has an outer cannula and an inner cannula. The advantage of an inner cannula, which can be locked into or out of place, is that it can slide in and out of the outer tube easily to facilitate cleaning and suctioning. The disadvantage is that there is a smaller internal diameter which may increase the work of breathing and actually trap secretions.

The tube may also be **cuffed** or **uncuffed**. A cuff is typically inflated with air or water and provides an airway seal and reduces aspiration or orotracheal secretions. Cuffs are typically used for patients requiring mechanical ventilation to prevent air leakage around the tube or in patients who have swallowing difficulties. The cuff is deflated when a patient no longer requires mechanical ventilation and is not aspirating. A patient with an inflated cuff would not use a speaking valve as this will not allow for airflow through the glottis (vocal cords).

A tracheostomy tube may also be **fenestrated** or **non-fenestrated**. A fenestrated tube has an additional opening in its back wall which permits upper airway airflow and facilitates speech. Fenestrated tubes may come with or without a cuff and are typically used for patients who are unable to tolerate a speaking valve.

Tracheostomy tubes come in a variety of shapes and sizes, and tube selection depends upon the patient. The dimensions of tracheostomy tubes are given by their inner diameter, outer diameter, length, and curvature. The inner and outer diameter sizes are marked on the flange of the tube. Tracheostomy tubes can be angled or curved, a feature that can be used to improve the fit of the tube in the trachea. Extra proximal length tubes facilitate placement in patients with large necks, and extra distal length tubes facilitate placement in patients with tracheal anomalies. When your physician chooses a size, considerations include lung health, upper airway resistance, airway clearance, trachea size and shape and communication/speech needs.

fig. 2

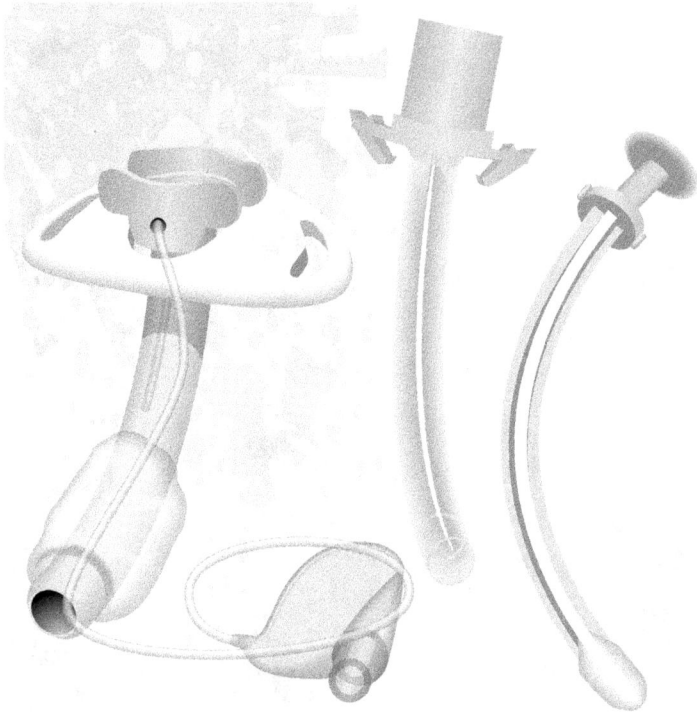

Cuffed tracheostomy tube with outer cannula (left), disposable inner cannula (middle), and obturators (right).

Part Four

Initial Aftercare

Once inserted, the tracheostomy tube is typically held in place with a soft, flexible tracheostomy tie or collar unless this is contraindicated due to a recent neck surgery. In this case, the tube may initially be sutured in place. Sutures are typically removed with the first tube change. The initial tracheostomy tube is usually changed 7-10 days after initial placement once the clinician is sure that the tract is well formed. In surgically performed tracheostomies, the tube can be changed as early as day 3-5 with appropriate precautions. A tracheostomy dressing, which is typically a small piece of gauze with a pre-made slit at the top, is often worn on the front of the neck under the tracheostomy tube flange and tie to prevent skin irritation.

> For a while after your tracheostomy, you may need to communicate with pen and paper. Once swelling improves and the tracheostomy site begins to heal, you may begin speaking. This will be discussed further later on.

Typically when you inhale, the nose acts to warm, humidify and filter the air you breathe. When a tracheostomy is created, you are breathing in and out of the hole in your neck, rather than your nose (unless the tracheostomy is capped). This means you are inhaling unfiltered cool, dry air directly into the trachea. This may cause drying and irritation of the tracheal mucosa as well as crusting of tracheal secretions.

In addition, the body produces extra mucus in the lungs and trachea to repel dust and other environmental irritants that normally would be filtered by the nose. To help you cope with dry air and to help thin tracheal secretions, humidification is used routinely in the initial post-procedure period. The humidification may be administered with or without oxygen (depending on your respiratory status), via a small mask that rests over your tracheostomy tube. The tracheostomy tube/stoma is suctioned with a flexible suction catheter any time there is visible or audible secretions in the airway. Your physician, nurse or caretaker will help you with suctioning.

If your tracheostomy tube has a dual cannula, the inner cannula is removed several times a day for cleaning. Recommendations on cleaning solutions vary. One method is to clean the inner cannula with a small brush and diluted hydrogen peroxide solution. The hospital staff will teach you when/how to suction your tracheostomy tube and how to clean the tube and the area around the stoma.

Part Five

Long-Term Aftercare

Some patients can have their tracheostomy removed (decannulated) before they are discharged from the hospital, but many patients have to go home with their tracheostomy tube. Understanding how to care for your tracheostomy appropriately, having necessary emergency supplies at home, and knowing how to monitor for signs of respiratory distress and signs of infection and skin breakdown will ease anxiety about the transition from hospital to home care. The case manager at the hospital will arrange delivery of necessary home equipment to take care of your tracheostomy once you are discharged. Prior to your discharge, be sure to ask your clinician which type, diameter and length of tracheostomy tube you have.

After discharge, you will need to schedule regular appointments with the physician who performed your tracheostomy to monitor for possible complications. You should call your doctor if you have difficulty breathing through the tube, bleeding through or around the tube, or pain, redness and/or swelling at the tracheostomy site. Recommendations for tracheostomy tube change vary and the first tube change will frequently occur within one week of initial placement. For patients with a need for long-term placement, tracheostomy tube change every 2-3 months is reasonable. This allows re-assessment of the soft tissue site on the neck and decreases the risk of bacterial colonization of the tube.

Once you are home, it is important to protect your airway from dust, bacteria and other environmental irritants. A tracheostomy cap (if permitted by your clinician) or a cloth tracheostomy bib may be used. Routine tracheostomy care should be performed at least once daily, but may be required more often as a result of mucus plugs or increased secretions.

A supply company will deliver materials to your home that are needed to care for your tracheostomy. This is usually arranged by your case manager before you leave the hospital.

Cleaning your tracheostomy tube and the area around the stoma at home requires the following supplies:

- Non-sterile gloves
- A sink
- Hydrogen peroxide
- Clean 4 x 4 fine mesh tracheostomy gauze pads
- Normal saline or tap water (Use distilled water if you have a septic tank or well water)
- Clean cotton-tipped swabs

- Clean pipe cleaners or small brush
- Clean washcloth
- Clean towel
- Tracheostomy tube ties
- Clean scissors

In addition to these cleaning supplies, you will probably have a suction kit and a humidification system delivered to your home.

These steps should be followed to clean the tracheostomy tube and the area around your stoma:

1. Wash your hands thoroughly with soap and water and sit in a comfortable position in front of a mirror.

2. Put on the gloves.

3. If your tube has an inner cannula, remove it. If you do not have an inner cannula, skip to the next step. Hold the inner cannula over a sink or basin and pour hydrogen peroxide over and into it. Use a pipe cleaner or small brush to clean the inner cannula. Thoroughly rinse with tap or distilled water then dry the inner cannula with clean fine mesh gauze. After suctioning the tracheostomy tube (see step 4), reinsert the inner cannula and lock into place.

4. Suction the tracheostomy tube. (This will be demonstrated by your clinician or nurse prior to discharge).

5. Remove and dispose of the soiled tracheostomy dressing around the neck. Inspect the skin around the stoma for redness, swelling, tenderness, drainage or lesions.

19

6. Soak the cotton tipped swabs in diluted hydrogen peroxide solution (50% water and 50% hydrogen peroxide). Use the swabs to clean the skin around the stoma and the external portion of the tracheostomy tube, including the neck flange.

7. Wet the wash cloth with normal saline, tap water or distilled water and wipe away the hydrogen peroxide and clean the skin.

8. Dry the exposed part of the tracheostomy tube and the skin around the stoma with a clean towel.

9. Change the tracheostomy tube ties making sure to hold the tracheostomy tube in place until the new tie is snug and secure. There should be no more than two fingers between the tie and your neck.

10. Place a clean tracheostomy gauze dressing under the tracheostomy tie and baseplate (flange).

11. Remove and dispose of your gloves and wash your hands.

Metal tracheostomy tubes, while less commonly used overall, are seen in the setting of patients that require long-term tracheostomy tube placement for chronic airway conditions. These tubes are reusable and typically have a lower profile that disposable tubes. *(See fig. 3 on next page)*

fig. 3

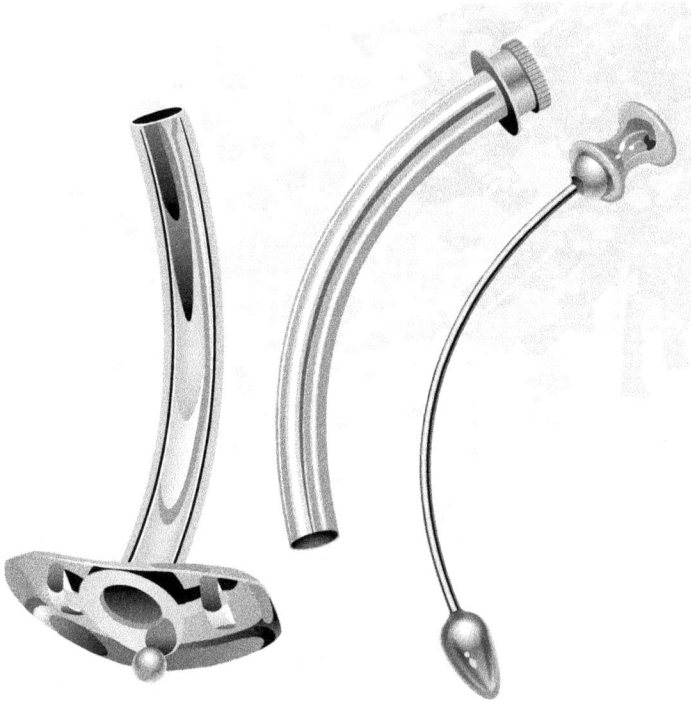

Metal tracheostomy tube with outer cannula (left), reusable inner cannula (middle), and obturator (right).

Part Six

Speech And Swallowing With A Tracheostomy Tube

When a tracheostomy tube is placed, the air flow to and from the lungs is redirected through the tracheostomy tube, instead of through the true vocal folds which consequently vibrate to produce sound (voicing). With this redirection of air through the tracheostomy tube, voicing is often lost. Speech Pathologists can work with patients in conjunction with their physicians to assist in restoring voice while the tracheostomy tube is in place.

In order to speak with a tracheostomy tube, airflow needs to be restored through the normal respiratory tract which includes the trachea, true vocal folds, mouth and nose. This is achieved in several ways including decreasing the size of the tracheostomy tube, changing to a cuffless tracheostomy tube, or using a type of tracheostomy tube with a hole in the back wall, known as a fenestration. *(See fig. 4 below)* Your physician will help determine the best type of tube for you based on your anatomy, current medical condition and future needs. Once there is sufficient airflow through the normal respiratory tract, a patient will be considered for a speaking valve.

fig. 4

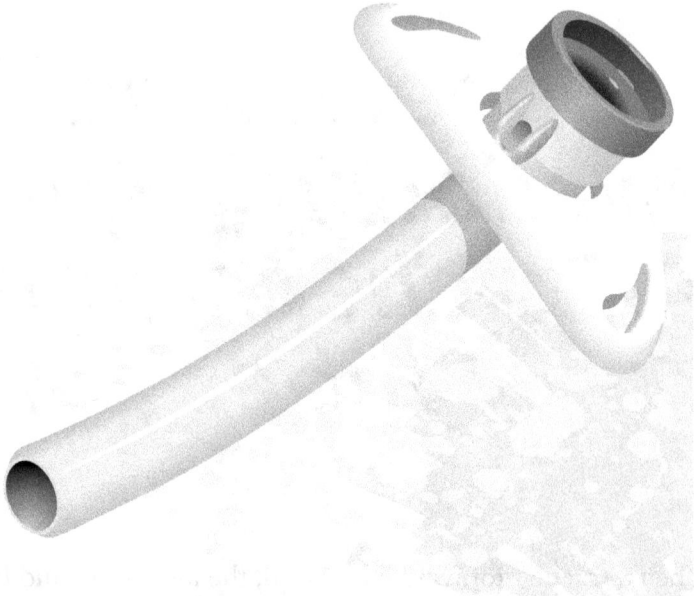

Uncuffed tracheostomy tube with 'screw on' decannulation plug in place (used to assist decannulation assessment).

A **speaking valve** is essentially a one way valve that is typically made of hard plastic and comes in a variety of shapes and colors. *(See fig. 5 on page 25)* The diameter of the speaking valve is universal and can fit on almost every size and brand of tracheostomy tube. Its color is determined by preference. For example, colored speaking valves are usually preferred in the hospital as they are easy to identify. On the other hand a white or clear valve which is less noticeable may be preferred once the patient is back home. Different shapes are also available to

fig. 5

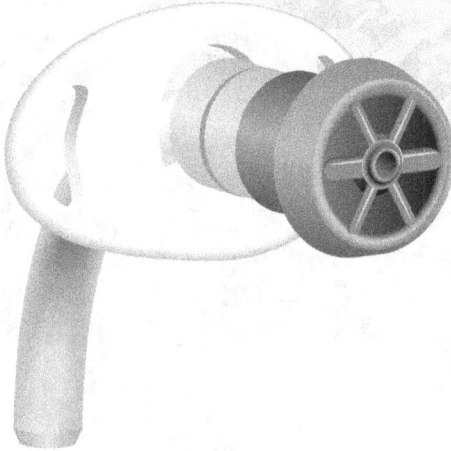

Uncuffed tracheostomy tube with speaking valve in place.

accommodate the patient's anatomy, finger dexterity, and vision. For example larger profile speaking valves may be helpful for patients with limited finger dexterity or decreased vision. A speech pathologist will assist the patient in determining the shape that is best for them.

Before a speaking valve is placed, the **speech pathologist** will make an assessment to determine the patient's abilities and physical condition. If a speaking valve is appropriate for the patient, it is placed on the end of the tracheostomy tube and pushed into place.

When a speaking valve is placed, inhalation continues as before, through the tracheostomy tube, mouth and nose. However, the exhaled air cannot escape through the tracheostomy tube because of the speaking valve. Rather it is directed through the normal respiratory tract including the true vocal folds, mouth and nose. This allows the vocal folds to vibrate and voicing is restored.

Some patients may experience difficulty breathing when the speaking valve is first put in place. This is natural as the body has to adjust to the air traveling a longer distance from the lungs to the mouth through the tracheostomy tube in the neck. Patients are usually encouraged to just sit and breathe as they adjust to the valve and the restoration of normal respiration. As they get used to this modified way of breathing, they can begin speaking. Over time, voicing will become natural and easy. If a patient is straining or experiencing excessive coughing, the speaking valve needs to be removed to allow the patient to catch their breath. When they are breathing normally again, the speaking valve can be put back in place.

Another common occurrence with a speaking valve is sputum production. Sputum is once again brought up into the mouth (oral cavity) with a forceful cough as opposed to being expectorated from the tracheostomy tube. This can seem frightening to the patient the first time it occurs, particularly if a tracheostomy tube has been in place for a long period of time before a speaking valve is placed. Sputum production is actually a positive sign and patients are encouraged to continue to cough and expectorate any sputum produced as they normally would. In some cases, patients may need to temporarily remove the speaking valve in order to successfully discharge all of the secretions.

A speaking valve should be worn as much as possible. This is a significant step toward capping the tracheostomy and hopefully decannulation (removal of the tracheostomy tube). The speaking valve should be removed at night if the patient is having any difficulty breathing, experiencing chest pain or tightness, or cannot successfully cough up thick sputum. It should only be cleaned with mild soap and warm water and allowed to dry overnight. Given the risk of aspiration a speaking valve should never be put on while wet.

It is also important to remember that the cuff of a cuffed tracheostomy tube should never be inflated when a speaking valve is worn. An inflated cuff will not allow adequate air to reach the nose and mouth to be exhaled.

Speaking valves are restorative. In addition to assisting in the normal restoration of exhalation, as mentioned above, they aid in the restoration of normal vocal fold movement which is necessary for both speaking and swallowing. They also provide improved hygiene as the tracheostomy tube is no longer wide open.

Part Seven

Decannulation

Decannulation is removal of the tracheostomy tube. Your physician will determine when it is appropriate for you to be decannulated. If you start with a large tracheostomy tube, downsizing of the tube is usually necessary prior to decannulation. The amount of time that a head and neck cancer patient requires a tracheostomy tube will vary from person to person. Prior to decannulation, you should be able to tolerate a cap on an uncuffed tube without any difficulty breathing. You should also have an effective cough when the tube is capped, meaning you are able to cough up and clear any respiratory secretions.

Similar to a speaking valve, a cap is a piece that is placed on the end of the tracheostomy tube. *(See fig. 6 on page 30)* However it does not allow any air to flow in or out of the tube. Therefore, when your tracheostomy is capped, you are breathing in and out through your nose and mouth, and the air is flowing through your trachea around the tracheostomy tube. Your physician may require a "capping trial" before decannulation. This usually means that you will need to breath comfortably with the tube capped for 24 hours continuously and without having to

fig. 6

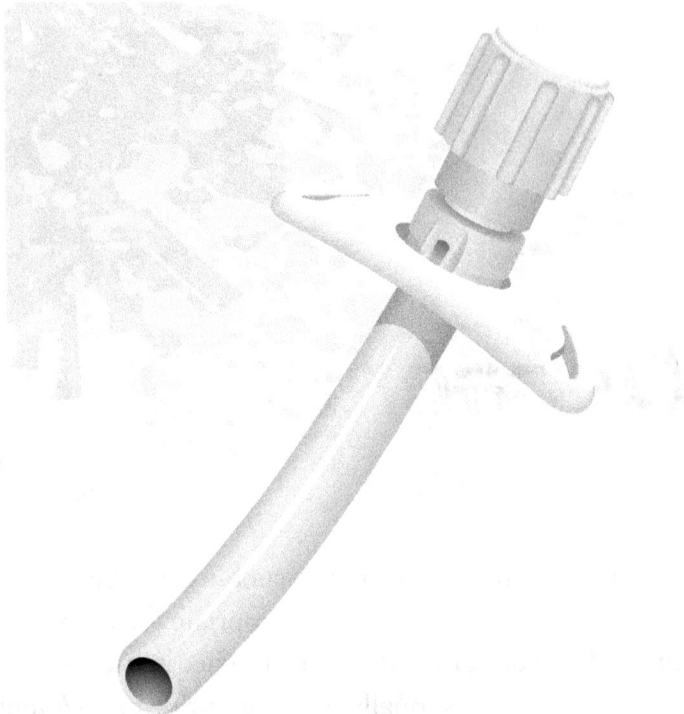

Uncuffed tracheostomy tube with decannulation cap in place (used to assist decannulation assessment)

suction the tracheostomy. Your physician may also perform a flexible laryngoscopic exam in clinic to confirm the resolution of any swelling in your throat and that your airway is patent without findings that would indicate an elevated risk of aspiration.

When your clinician determines it is safe to decannulate, he or she will remove the tracheostomy tie and slide the tracheostomy tube out from the tract. This is a relatively painless procedure. The area around the stoma is cleaned. The stoma site is dressed with an airtight dressing which should be changed daily (or more frequently if needed) until the stoma has closed completely.

to physician. A small layer of xeroform petroleum gauze may be placed over the stoma, covered by a slightly larger clean gauze dressing. This is taped on all four sides to prevent air leakage. When you speak or cough, you should apply pressure to the dressing over the stoma to prevent air escape. Persistent leakage of air through the stoma will prolong stoma healing.

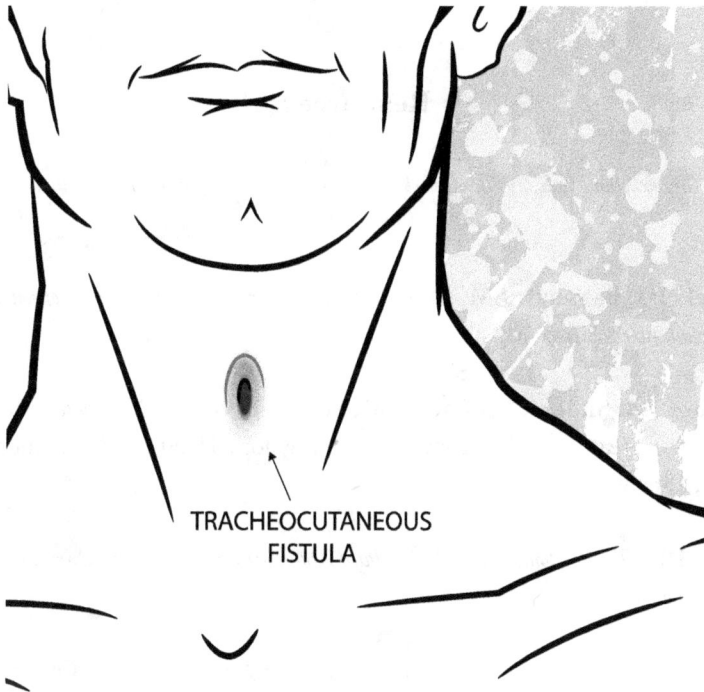

fig. 7

TRACHEOCUTANEOUS
FISTULA

Tracheocutaneous fistula at the site of prior tracheostomy.

You may be able to transition from an airtight dressing to a band-aid in the final days of healing. The time it takes the tracheostomy stoma to heal also varies from person to person.

It typically takes about 1-2 weeks for the stoma to close completely. Patients with a history of radiation to the neck or with chronic diseases, such as diabetes, may take longer.

Sometimes you may have an external overgrowth of granulation tissue at the tracheostomy site. This is red, healing tissue. Excess granulation tissue can be chemically cauterized by your physician to promote healing. Uncommonly, patients develop a tracheocutaneous fistula, which means the stoma does not close completely. *(See fig. 7 on page 31)* A relatively minor outpatient surgical procedure may be required to close this.

Resources

http://my.clevelandclinic.org/head_neck/patients/head_neck_cancer/tracheostomy_care. aspx

Engels PT, Bagshaw SM, Meier M, et al. *Tracheostomy: From Insertion To Decannulation.* Canadian Journal of Surgery 2009; 52:427-433.

Garner JM, Shoemaker-Moyle M, Franzese CB. *Adult Outpatient Tracheostomy Care: Practices And Perspectives.* Otolaryngology-Head and Neck Surgery 2007; 136: 301-306.

Hess DR. *Tracheostomy Tubes And Related Appliances.* Respiratory Care 2005; 50(4): 497-510.

Mitchell RB, et al. *Clinical Consensus Statement: Tracheostomy Care.* Otolaryngology-Head and Neck Surgery 2013; 148:6-20.

Notes

Notes

About The Authors

Kara Mosesso, ANP-BC: *Survivorship Nurse Practitioner, Memorial Sloan Kettering Cancer Center:* Kara Mosesso received her BA in Social Science at Providence College. She went on to obtain her Masters of Science in Nursing (MSN) at Boston College and subsequently worked for four years as the outpatient Head and Neck cancer Nurse Practitioner in the Department of Otolaryngology-Head and Neck Surgery at Tufts Medical Center. Currently, she is the Survivorship Nurse Practitioner for allogeneic stem cell transplant patients at Memorial Sloan Kettering Cancer Center. In addition she is a clinical instructor for the Tufts University School of Medicine Physician Assistant Program.

Elizabeth Von Euw, MS, CCC-SLP: *Speech Language Pathologist, Tufts Medical Center:* Elizabeth Von Euw received both her Bachelor of Science and Masters of Science in the field of Speech Language Pathology at Northeastern University. She is currently licensed by the American Speech-Language-Hearing Association (ASHA) as well as the commonwealth of Massachusetts. Upon graduation, Elizabeth worked in a private practice working between two acute care hospitals in addition to a long term care health facility before transitioning to Tufts Medical Center. Over the past ten years Elizabeth has worked closely with multiple disciplines in the acute care setting with a focus on swallowing evaluation and intervention. Being part of an academic medical center, she has provided multiple lectures to the medical staff, local colleges and actively supervises local graduate students in the field of Speech Language Pathology.

Miriam O'Leary, MD: *Assistant Professor, Department of Otolaryngology Head & Neck Surgery, Tufts Medical Center:* Dr. O'Leary received her BA at Rosemont College and her medical degree at the University of Connecticut School of Medicine. She completed a residency in otolaryngology – head and neck surgery at Boston University, and a fellowship in head and neck surgery and microvascular reconstruction at the University of Miami. She is an Assistant Professor in the Department of Otolaryngology – Head and Neck Surgery at Tufts Medical Center, practicing extirpative and reconstructive head and neck surgery.

Richard O. Wein, MD, FACS: *Associate Professor, Department of Otolaryngology Head & Neck Surgery, Tufts Medical Center:* Dr. Wein performed his residency in Otolaryngology-Head & Neck Surgery at the University of Rochester Medical Center in Rochester, NY. He subsequently completed fellowship in Head & Neck Surgical Oncology and Microvascular Reconstruction at the University of Pennsylvania Health System in Philadelphia, PA. He is currently an Associate Professor in the Department of Otolaryngology – Head & Neck Surgery at Tufts Medical Center and a Faculty Advisor at the Tufts University School of Medicine in Boston, MA. His practice and research interest are focused on the multidisciplinary management of head and neck cancer and the surgical treatment of thyroid, salivary and advanced skin neoplasms.

www.ingramcontent.com/pod-product-compliance
Lightning Source LLC
Chambersburg PA
CBHW060530280326
41933CB00014B/3125